FAST FACTS

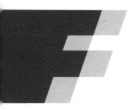

MX 0537391 3

Superficial Fungal Infections

Indispensable

Guides to

Clinical

Practice

M lcoln ᴿⁱ

Seruor Lecture.,   . ᴊl Myᴄ
Mycology Unit, Department of
Bacteriology and Immunology,
Haartman Institute, Helsinki, Finland

Boni Elewski
Professor of Dermatology,
Department of Dermatology,
University of Alabama, Birmingham,
Alabama, USA

D1448438

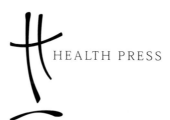

HEALTH PRESS

Oxford

Fast Facts – Superficial Fungal Infections
First published 2000

Text © 2000 Malcolm Richardson, Boni Elewski
© 2000 in this edition Health Press Limited
Health Press Limited, Elizabeth House, Queen Street, Abingdon,
Oxford OX14 3JR, UK
Tel: +44 (0)1235 523233
Fax: +44 (0)1235 523238

Fast Facts is a trade mark of Health Press Limited.

The publisher and the authors have made every effort to ensure the
accuracy of this book, but cannot accept responsibility for any errors
or omissions.

In addition to our own original work, some of the illustrations have
originated from other sources. We would like to take this opportunity
to thank our friends and colleagues, both past and present, for their
generosity in making them available to us.

A CIP catalogue record for this title is available from the British Library.

ISBN 1-899541-76-4

Richardson, M (Malcolm)
Fast Facts – Superficial Fungal Infections/
Malcolm Richardson, Boni Elewski

Printed by Fine Print (Services) Ltd, Oxford, UK

Introduction   5

Common fungi and their routes
of transmission   7

Laboratory diagnosis   13

Tinea capitis   23

Tinea corporis and cruris   30

Tinea unguium (onychomycosis)   35

Other tinea infections   41

Pityriasis versicolor   45

Cutaneous *Candida* infections   49

Future trends   52

Key references   53

Index   54

Introduction

Superficial fungal infections (dermatomycoses) are very common and occur throughout the world. Most of these infections are caused by dermatophytic moulds (the terms tinea and ringworm are synonymous with dermatomycosis). Dermatophytic infections are contagious diseases caused by either a human (anthropophilic) or animal (zoophilic) species of dermatophyte fungi.

A second group of superficial infections is caused by yeasts. *Candida* species cause infections of the mucous membranes, skin and fingernails (candidiasis or thrush) and *Malassezia furfur* (*Pityrosporum orbiculare*) infects the skin, usually the trunk (pityriasis versicolor). Both organisms are commensals of humans.

These infections can be difficult to diagnose and are often mistaken for other disorders, such as eczema or psoriasis. With the exception of nail infections, fungal infections respond quickly and can be managed effectively if treated correctly. In *Fast Facts – Superficial Fungal Infections*, we have tried to provide clinicians with a brief, accessible and illustrated introduction to fungal diseases of the skin, hair and nails. Particular attention has been paid to clinical presentation, laboratory investigation, diagnosis, treatment and prevention. A special effort has been made to ensure that dosage recommendations are accurate and in agreement with consensus opinion at the time of publication. The medications described do not necessarily have specific approval by the appropriate regulatory authorities for use as they are recommended here. As dosage regimens may be modified as new research and laboratory studies are undertaken, clinicians are advised to check packaging information for recommended doses and contraindications for use. This is particularly important with new or infrequently used drugs.

CHAPTER 1
Common fungi and their routes of transmission

Fungal infections of the skin, hair and nails are among the most common causes of skin disease in the UK and USA. They can be difficult to diagnose, however, and are often mistaken for other disorders, such as eczema or psoriasis. With the exception of nail infections, fungal infections respond quickly and can be managed satisfactorily if treated correctly.

Fungal infections are generally diagnosed on the basis of clinical appearance. However, the steroid response of a dermatosis may be used in diagnosis, so it is important that appropriate investigations are instigated before administering any form of treatment, which often comprises an antifungal/steroid cream. This approach will enable the diagnosis to be reassessed if initial treatment is unsuccessful.

The principal fungal infections are caused by dermatophyte fungi (tinea or ringworm infections), and the yeasts *Candida albicans* and *Pityrosporum orbiculare* (*Malassezia furfur*).

Dermatophytes

Dermatophytes belong to three genera:
- *Trichophyton*
- *Microsporum*
- *Epidermophyton*.

Aetiology. Dermatophytes are characterized by their ability to exist and grow in keratin. This enables them to invade the stratum corneum of the skin and keratinized structures, such as hair and nails, with minimal stimulation of the host's immune response.

Fungal growth in keratinized tissues is restricted to the production of hyphae, which branch and segment into chains of spores called arthrospores or arthroconidia (Figure 1.1). Arthrospores are the main means of dissemination and propagation of the fungus (Figures 1.2–1.5), and can remain viable and infective in the environment and exfoliated skin for many months, and even years. Although arthrospores are common, in the horny layer of the skin and in nail, hyphae may be present without

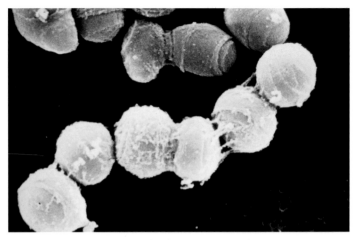

Figure 1.1 Arthrospores of *Trichophyton mentagrophytes.*

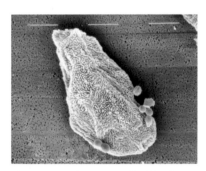

Figure 1.2 Arthrospores of *Trichophyton mentagrophytes* adhering to a human corneocyte.

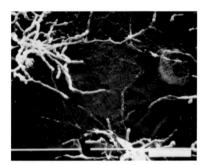

Figure 1.3 Growth of *Trichophyton mentagrophytes* on human stratum corneum.

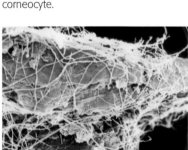

Figure 1.4 Growth of *Trichophyton mentagrophytes* on human nail.

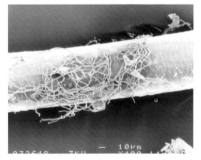

Figure 1.5 Growth of *Trichophyton mentagrophytes* on a human hair shaft.

arthrospore formation, irrespective of the species involved. In hair, the type and extent of invasion varies according to the species of fungus, and this affects the presenting clinical symptoms. The hyphae and arthrospores of certain species of dermatophytes remain strictly within the hair shaft (endothrix), while others form a sheath of arthrospores around the outside of the shaft (ectothrix). In endothrix infection, the hair shaft is almost completely destroyed and breaks off at, or below, the mouth of the follicle; in ectothrix infection, the hair remains sufficiently robust to stay intact to a length of 2–3 mm above the mouth of the follicle. The variations in the form of hair invasion are not specific, however, and, as with infections of skin and nail, culture is required to identify the species of fungus causing the infection.

Species. The ringworm fungi that normally infect man are the most highly specialized group of dermatophytes. They rarely infect lower animals and often show a strong preference for a particular body part, only occasionally being found in other regions; for example, *Microsporum audouinii* infects scalp hair, but is seldom found on skin.

There are about 40 recognized species of dermatophytes. Some are only able to infect man (anthropophilic), whereas others are primarily animal pathogens (zoophilic), but can also infect man. A few species are found as saprhrophytes in soil (geophilic), and cause sporadic infections in both man and animals. Most infections in the UK and USA are produced by six species:

- *Trichophyton rubrum*
- *Trichophyton interdigitale* (also known as *Trichophyton mentagrophytes* var. *interdigitale*; Figure 1.6)
- *Trichophyton mentagrophytes* (also known as *Trichophyton mentagrophytes* var. *mentagrophytes*)
- *Trichophyton verrucosum*
- *Microsporum canis* (Figure 1.7)
- *Epidermophyton floccosum* (Figure 1.8).

Transmission

Animal to man. Many dermatophytes are transmitted to man through contact with an infected animal. Up to 50% of human ringworm infections

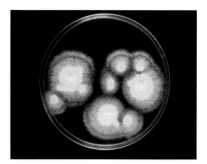

Figure 1.6 Culture of *Trichophyton mentagrophytes* showing typical floccose colonies that become cream coloured and powdery in the centre.

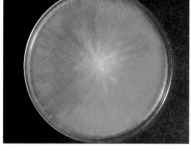

Figure 1.7 Culture of *Microsporum canis* which has a flat surface that becomes lemon-yellow with age.

Figure 1.8 Culture of *Epidermophyton floccosum* showing the typical khaki-coloured appearance. As the culture ages, the surface may become folded and white floccose patches appear.

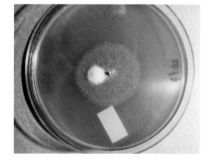

are contracted from animals, particularly in rural areas. Examples include:

- *T. verrucosum* from infected cattle, which causes pustular tinea barbae and tinea corporis lesions in man (Figure 1.9)
- *M. canis* from infected dogs and cats, which causes tinea capitis and tinea corporis (Figures 1.10 and 1.11)
- *T. mentagrophytes* from infected rodents
- *Trichophyton erinacea* from infected hedgehogs, which is rare but does occur (Figure 1.12)
- *Trichophyton equinum* from infected horses, which is also rare (Figure 1.13).

The organisms are transmitted to man primarily through direct or indirect contact with other infected humans or animals. Infection can follow direct or indirect contact with infected scales or hairs. The chances of successful transmission are enhanced by the prolonged viability of dermatophyte

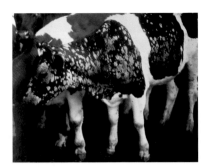

Figure 1.9 Cattle ringworm due to *Trichophyton verrucosum*.

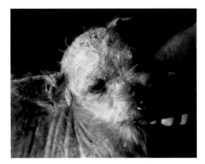

Figure 1.10 Ringworm due to *Microsporum canis* in a dog.

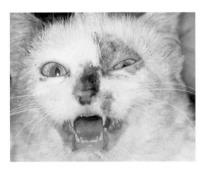

Figure 1.11 Ringworm due to *Microsporum canis* in a cat.

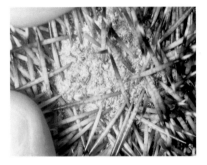

Figure 1.12 Ringworm due to *Trichophyton erinacea* in a hedgehog.

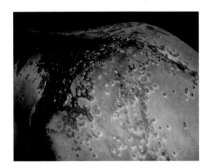

Figure 1.13 Ringworm due to *Trichophyton equinum* in a horse.

arthroconidia in exfoliated and traumatized skin. Children are more susceptible to infection than adults.

Atypical dermatophyte infection. Although, as a general rule, dermatophytes do not invade below the keratin layer they may occasionally do so

11

in specific circumstances, usually when the patient is immunosuppressed. Granulomatous or mycetoma-like lesions can develop in such cases, but they are rarely seen.

The alteration of a simple dermatophyte infection secondary to the long-term use of topical steroids is much more common. It is often referred to as tinea incognito, but this term tends to add legitimacy to a situation where the disease is misdiagnosed and mistreated. In such cases the integrity of the ring-like edge is lost, the scaling disappears and small nodules develop. The disease looks less and less like a fungal infection, which often compounds the vicious circle of misdiagnosis and mistreatment.

Yeasts

Superficial infections caused by yeasts are predominantly due to the genus *Candida*, in particular *C. albicans*. These organisms are common commensals of the mouth, gastrointestinal tract, vagina and, to a lesser extent, the skin.

Another yeast that infects the skin is *P. orbiculare* (*M. furfur*), which causes pityriasis (tinea) versicolor. Transmission of yeast infections is both between individuals and intraindividual.

Scytalidium dimidiatum infection

This non-dermatophyte mould does merit separate consideration. It is the only non-dermatophyte mould that is a true pathogen of both skin and nail, and in some parts of South-East Asia this organism is the commonest cause of tinea pedis. It is primarily a geophilic plant pathogen and produces black discoloration of the nail plate. It is important to recognize the possibility of such infection, as its growth in culture will be suppressed by antibacterial agents added to the medium. It is to be hoped that this pathogen will not become significantly more prevalent as it does not respond well to any known antifungal agents.

CHAPTER 2
Laboratory diagnosis

Clinical criteria provide only a presumptive diagnosis of fungal infection. Characteristic lesions often strongly suggest a fungal aetiology, although the lesions may resemble those of other diseases. Furthermore, their appearance is frequently atypical because of previous therapy with, for example, topical steroids.

Role of the laboratory
Laboratory procedures provide information that enables clinicians to confirm a clinical diagnosis, establish a fungal cause of a disease of unknown aetiology or exclude fungal involvement when there are several possible diagnoses. When a fungal infection has been diagnosed, the laboratory can help select and monitor antifungal therapy, follow the subsequent course of the disease, and confirm a mycological cure.

Objectives. The main objective of the laboratory is the efficient and rapid detection and recovery of fungi from clinical specimens, and the subsequent accurate identification of any fungal isolates. Laboratory diagnosis should always be employed prior to the institution of treatment because dermatophytes, non-dermatophyte moulds and yeasts respond differently to antifungal agents. There are two key points.
• Is the skin condition caused by a fungus?
• What is the causal agent?

Clinical and laboratory cooperation. Cooperation between the clinician and the laboratory is essential to ensure that an accurate diagnosis is made and appropriate treatment initiated as early as possible. Specimens must be taken properly, and information about the patient must be given succinctly and precisely. Details about the patient must include:
• the age and sex of the patient (sex is particularly important in the case of cutaneous yeast infections)
• the part of the body from which the specimen was taken
• contact with animals

- clinical history and preliminary diagnosis.

The patient's history may be particularly important; for example, immuno-suppressant drugs can enable saprophytic fungi to become pathogenic, while knowledge of the patient's native country or travel abroad may include an exotic mycosis.

The success of laboratory diagnosis is determined by the expertise of the laboratory staff and by the quality of the sample sent for examination. Material should be sent to a medical mycology laboratory that is experienced in the diagnosis of fungal infections. Although there are relatively few specialist laboratories, they should be used in preference to local bacteriology laboratories with no experience in fungal diagnostic techniques.

A laboratory diagnosis may be made in two ways:

- demonstration of the fungus in a specimen on microscopy; this may confirm or eventually lead to the correct clinical diagnosis
- culture of the fungus, which will allow specific identification and assist in the choice of treatment.

Microscopy

Collection of specimens. Lesions of the skin, scalp and nail should be cleansed with surgical spirit or 70% alcohol before samples are collected; this improves the chances of detecting the fungus microscopically. Cleansing is essential if greasy ointments, creams or powders have been applied to the sample site. Obviously, specimens should not be taken after a topical antifungal preparation has been applied, as this is likely to affect fungal growth.

Skin, hair and nail samples should be collected into folded squares of stiff black paper, which when secured with a paper clip are suitable for sending through the mail and several samples can be placed in the same envelope. The use of black paper allows the specimen to dry out, which helps to reduce bacterial contamination, and provides conditions under which specimens can be conveniently stored for long periods without any appreciable loss in viability of the fungus. Furthermore, laboratory staff can process and conserve the specimen without transferring it to another vehicle.

Black paper envelopes specifically designed for the collection and transportation of skin, hair and nail samples are extremely convenient (Figure 2.1); they are available from Dermaco Ltd (PO Box 470,

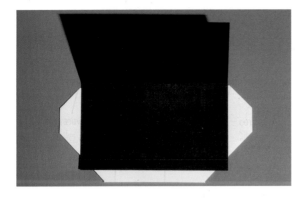

Figure 2.1 Dermapak – commercial skin sample collecting and packaging envelope.

Toddington, Bedfordshire, LU5 6BF, UK) and Key Scientific Products (149C Texas Avenue, Round Rock, Texas 78664, USA). The use of screw-capped bottles, plastic containers or glass slides secured with adhesive tape for transportation of specimens has a number of disadvantages; the sample has to be transferred before processing, and it is often difficult to find and remove small fragments of material from large containers. Furthermore, postage of such containers is expensive.

Quality of specimen

Skin. In glabrous skin, the advancing edge of the lesion provides the most satisfactory specimen. Material from skin lesions should be collected by scraping outwards from the edges of the lesion with a blunt scalpel blade held perpendicular to the skin. With infection of the toe-webs, the soggy skin should be peeled away. If vesicles are present, the whole top of the lesion should be removed.

Scalp. Hair from areas of suspected infection must be submitted with the root end. It should be plucked not clipped. Only the first 5–6 mm of hair are of any value in most instances. Samples can also be taken by brushing the scalp with a hairbrush; the skin scales can be cultured directly (Figure 2.2). In the case of 'black-dot' tinea capitis lesions in which the hair shafts have broken off, the affected area must be scraped with a scalpel as with skin infections.

Nail. If possible, the specimen should not include the distal edge. The affected nail should be clipped as proximally as possible through the entire thickness of the nail, taking care to obtain the maximum amount of crumbly material. This material is concentrated on the underside of the nail, where

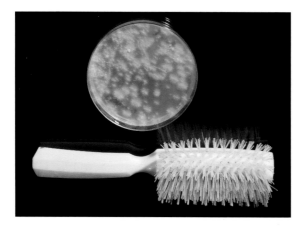

Figure 2.2 After passing through the hair, the brush is tapped over the surface of a laboratory culture medium.

the nail is most thickened, and a small pair of scissors is therefore useless for sampling purposes; the use of a pincer-type nail clipper of adequate size is most effective. Subungual debris is only occasionally useful and, if included, should be submitted as a separate specimen.

When nail dystrophy is wholly proximal, it is not possible to obtain a specimen by clipping. In such cases, a scraping can be taken from the affected portion of the nail with a scalpel blade. Alternatively, material can be obtained by the use of a small biopsy punch, but care must be taken not to cause pain by penetrating the nail. Fungi can then be visualized and isolated from the biopsy specimens. However, as this technique requires a local anaesthetic and special expertise, it is not a practical diagnostic method.

Candida can be isolated from beneath the lateral nail fold by running a bacteriology swab dipped in sterile saline along the length of the fold. The swab can then be replaced in its holder and sent to the laboratory. The swab should be processed as soon as possible, because the viability of the yeast will be adversely affected if it is allowed to dry out. This problem can be avoided by transporting the specimen in plain transport medium.

Alternatively, a disposable plastic loop can be passed underneath the nail fold where the cuticle is detached and rubbed directly onto a culture plate. This requires special facilities, however, which are not generally available.

Quantity of specimen. As fungal elements are not particularly numerous, or equally distributed, the quantity as well as the quality of the specimen taken is important. As a general rule, attempts should be made to obtain 10–15 mm^2

of skin, about twice this amount of nail, and 4–6 hair bases. This is sufficient to allow satisfactory microscopic examination and culture. A diagnosis can often be made using less material, but there will always be doubts about a negative result if less than 10 fragments of specimen are processed for culture, and an adequate microscopic examination cannot be made.

Request forms and results

Request forms are designed to ensure that all the essential information (i.e. name, age, sex, sample site) is supplied. Any relevant additional information (e.g. animal contacts, residence or foreign travel) is often helpful. It is also important to ensure that the name and address of the person to whom the report should be sent is provided.

In most laboratories, microscopic examination is carried out on the day that the specimen is received and a positive result is notified on that day. A culture result should be given as soon as it is available (usually within 10–14 days); negative results after 21 days. If clinical doubt persists after receiving a negative laboratory report, a further specimen should be sent to the laboratory.

Demonstration of the fungus. It is relatively easy to demonstrate the presence of a fungus by microscopy, because the filaments and yeast forms of fungi are sufficiently large to be recognized. Occasionally, the morphology is characteristic and the fungus can be identified without culture (e.g. the hyphae and yeast cells of *M. furfur*, and the conidia of *Scopulariopsis brevicaulis*; see Table 2.2). The three principal methods of examining clinical specimens for fungi are:

- direct examination – a simple technique that has gained popularity and is particularly suitable when scanty fungus is present and/or the operator is relatively inexperienced
- examination of a Gram-stained smear from a swab on a slide
- examination of histological sections.

Microscopical examination is an important preliminary procedure which can indicate the pathogen involved. The principal advantage of direct microscopy is the speed with which the results can be obtained and, in turn, a presumptive diagnosis made. Occasionally, therapy may be started on the basis of the direct microscopy results.

The sensitivity and specificity of microscopy depends on three main factors: the number of organisms present in the specimen, the type of fungus and the expertise of the observer. The ability to differentiate between fungal structures and artefacts in the sample increases with experience. Identification of a fungus by its morphology in skin, nail and hair is, however, usually impossible, though exceptions include M. *furfur* in skin, and S. *brevicaulis* in nail.

Processing of specimens. Specimens of skin, nail and hair need to be digested in a solution of potassium hydroxide so that the tissue layers are thin enough to enable the hyphae or other fungal elements to be seen (Table 2.1). In the case of skin and nail, random samples should be taken from several pieces of the material provided. When tinea capitis is suspected, hair may be examined under a Wood's lamp, a specialized lamp that produces ultraviolet radiation at a wavelength of 366 nm. Bright green fluorescence is characteristic of *Microsporum* infection, while dull green fluorescence is typical of favus. Infections caused by common *Trichophyton* species such as *Trichophyton tonsurans* and *Trichophyton violaceum*

TABLE 2.1

Processing of tissue specimens for direct microscopy

- Hold the material with a pair of forceps and use a scalpel to chop the sample into small fragments

- Place a drop of 20% potassium hydroxide solution onto a microscope slide. Moisten the tip of a mounted needle in the drop, and pick up and place several small fragments of specimen into the solution

- Place a coverslip on top of the drop and allow to stand for 30 minutes; nail clippings should be allowed to stand for 2–3 hours, or overnight in a humid chamber

- Using the upper surface of the thumbnail, or the base of a wooden pencil, press the coverslip gently several times to flatten the tissue into a single layer of cells

- View the slide under low-power microscopy initially and carefully scan the entire specimen, and then view anything of interest under high power

do not fluoresce. Any parts that fluoresce should be selected for microscopic examination.

Staining procedures for keratinous tissue are generally time consuming or unsatisfactory, giving poor differentiation of the fungal elements. The exceptions are the Parker's ink and Calcofluor white staining procedures.

- The Parker's ink procedure involves adding the blue-black ink to the potassium hydroxide 20% to produce a 1% solution, and then introducing the specimen. When interpreting results, it is important to remember that artefacts can also take up the stain.

- Calcofluor white fluoresces on exposure to ultraviolet light. The procedure involves adding one drop of 0.1% Calcofluor white (Sigma) containing 0.05% Evan's blue to one drop of 20% potassium hydroxide solution and then introducing the stain to the specimen. The slide should be allowed to stand for 30 minutes before being viewed under a fluorescence microscope using the blue light.

Interpretation of results

Essentially, three groups of fungi can invade the keratinous layer, namely:

- ringworm fungi (dermatophytes)
- yeasts
- other moulds (mycelial fungi, often darkly pigmented).

The observation of fungal elements in keratinous tissue is presumptive evidence of a fungal infection (Table 2.2). This confirms the clinical diagnosis and may enable antifungal therapy to be instigated. Conversely, careful microscopical examination, which excludes a fungal infection, can contribute greatly to the overall management of a patient.

Hair infections are exclusively caused by dermatophytes, except in the clinical conditions known as black and white piedras. Both of these conditions occur in tropical climates, though white piedras are occasionally found in temperate zones. White piedra is a fungal infection of the hair of the scalp, beard and moustache, and sometimes pubic areas, characterized by soft greyish-white nodules. These are of variable consistency and arranged in rows along the hair shaft to which they are adherent. Black piedra is also a hair disease, which is characterized by the appearance of dark brown or black nodules. These are gritty and adhere to the distal third of the hair.

TABLE 2.2

Characteristic microscopical features of fungi

- Fungal hyphae appear as branched colourless filaments that pass unhindered through the cell walls of the host tissue. The hyphae of ringworm fungi, however, often disintegrate into arthrospores (a)

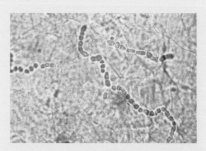

(a) Microscopical appearance of infected skin scrapings mounted in potassium hydroxide.

- The presence of colourless hyphae or hyphae with a faint greenish tinge disintegrating into chains of arthrospores generally indicates a dermatophyte infection

- In pityriasis, specimens stained with Parker's ink show a 'bananas and grapes' appearance, characteristic of the causal organism (*M. furfur*). Staining with Calcofluor white is very effective (b). An abundance of short, slightly curved hyphae indicates pityriasis versicolor

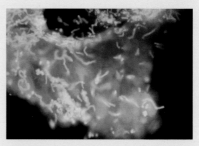

(b) Microscopical appearance of *Malassezia furfur* using Calcofluor white.

- Budding yeast cells and pseudohyphae confirm the clinical diagnosis of a yeast infection. *Candida* is recognized by the appearance of blastoconidia and pseudo-hyphae either in potassium hydroxide-digested specimens or in Calcofluor white-stained material (c)

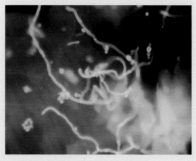

(c) Microscopical appearance of *Candida albicans* in infected skin scrapings using Calcofluor white stain.

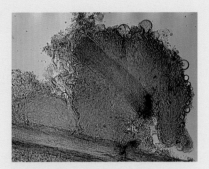

(d) Ectothrix invasion of hair by *Microsporum canis*.

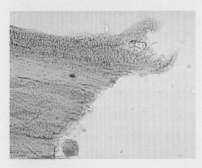

(e) Endothrix invasion of hair by *Trichophyton tonsurans*.

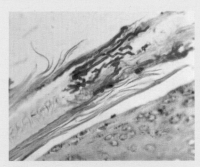

(f) Invasion of a hair follicle by *Microsporum canis* stained with periodic acid-Schiff.

- Hair should be examined very carefully as few hyphae may be present in infected material. Arthrospores are, however, produced in abundance, and may be seen along the outside (endothrix) (d) or within the hair shaft (ectothrix) (e). Histopathological staining of infected hair follicles will also reveal fungal elements (f)

- Other mycelial fungi (e.g. *Scytalidium*) can take on various forms in tissue and can be difficult to distinguish from *Candida* hyphae and from dermatophytes, particularly if dermatophytes have been subjected to antifungal treatment. They do, however, tend to produce narrow, hyaline hyphae that often vary in width; in the broader parts, the cell contents appear to withdraw from the cell membrane giving a double-contoured appearance

Culture of the fungus

In order to identify the pathogen, it is necessary to culture the sample (Figures 2.3 and 2.4). When fungi in tissue are not numerous or fungal elements are not viable, as is often the case, a large amount of specimen should be inoculated on laboratory culture media. The interpretation of a mixture of fungal colonies from nail specimens in particular requires specialist knowledge (Figure 2.5).

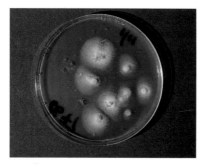

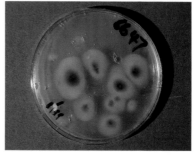

Figure 2.3 *Trichophyton rubrum* culture from infected skin (upper surface appearance of colony) showing white floccose colonies with a heaped centre.

Figure 2.4 *Trichophyton rubrum* culture from infected skin (reverse appearance of culture) showing the characteristic dark-brown pigmentation.

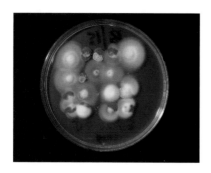

Figure 2.5 Mixed culture appearance of *Trichophyton rubrum*, non-dermatophytes and yeasts.

CHAPTER 3

Tinea capitis

Tinea capitis is a common infection occurring predominantly in prepubertal children. Although infection in adults can occur, it is rare. One risk factor for adult disease is immunosuppression resulting from drugs or therapeutic interventions. *Microsporum* and *Trichophyton* species are the aetiological agents of tinea capitis. The most common causative fungi are *T. tonsurans* and *M. canis*.

All species can cause similar types of infection in terms of inflammatory and non-inflammatory conditions. However, the organisms that cause endothrix tinea capitis are *T. tonsurans*, *T. violaceum*, *Trichophyton soudense*, *Trichophyton gourvilli* and, occasionally, *T. rubrum*.

The fluorescent *Microsporum* species (*M. canis*, *M. audouinii*, *Microsporum ferrugineum* and *Microsporum distortum*) and other *Trichophyton* organisms, such as *T. rubrum*, which can also cause endothrix infection, and *T. mentagrophytes*, produce ectothrix infection.

Epidemiology

Although the epidemiology of tinea capitis has changed over the past 30 years, the infection remains endemic in the developing world and mainly involves anthropophilic species. Anthropophilic infection secondary to *M. audouinii* is now relatively uncommon in the developed world as a result of improved social conditions and the development of effective treatments. Sporadic cases of *M. canis* infection occur worldwide and are difficult to eradicate, because domestic animals, such as cats and dogs, are the primary hosts.

More recently, the prevalence of *T. tonsurans* has increased significantly, particularly in poor urban communities. The infection is more common in individuals of African descent, though the reasons for this are unclear. *T. tonsurans* is also the most common pathogen in the USA and is emerging as such in Europe. It is likely that both hair-care products and genetic predisposition play a role in susceptibility to this infection.

23

Clinical presentation

Tinea capitis can present in several different ways. The clinical picture varies geographically, and is also dependent on the primary host. Tinea capitis normally presents as either grey-patch ringworm, usually associated with *M. audouinii* and previously common in North America and Europe, or as black-dot ringworm, often associated with *T. tonsurans* or *T. violaceum* infection. Lesions vary from a dry, scaly patch of alopecia, often associated with *M. audouinii* or *M. canis*, to a kerion, which is most commonly seen in *T. tonsurans* or *T. verrucosum* infection. *T. tonsurans* also produces a more diffuse infection, resulting in fragile broken hairs.

Alopecia. The most common presentation is as a discrete patch of alopecia, with or without scale (Figures 3.1 and 3.2), that may mimic alopecia areata. Patients with tinea capitis also develop posterior cervical adenopathy, which helps to distinguish tinea capitis from other cutaneous diseases that result in alopecia, such as alopecia areata. Broken hairs close to the root in the scalp may also be seen and, if the patient has black hair, this is often referred to as a 'black-dot' presentation. Black dots may occur within a single patch or diffusely across the scalp.

Kerion. The development of pustules and abscesses, known as a kerion, is another possible presentation (Figure 3.3). Such abscesses can be painful and several centimetres in diameter. A kerion is an advanced form of tinea capitis and is a hypersensitive reaction. It can occur on some parts of the scalp,

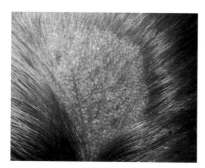

Figure 3.1 Tinea capitis caused by *Trichophyton tonsurans*, the main cause in the USA.

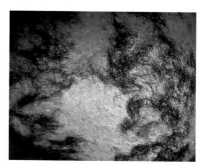

Figure 3.2 Tinea capitis caused by *Trichophyton tonsurans*.

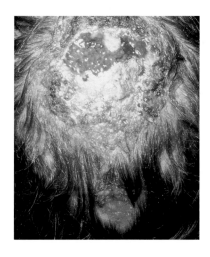

Figure 3.3 A kerion is the most extreme type of inflammatory lesion seen in tinea capitis, and forms a boggy and pustular mass. Hair loss is seldom permanent unless an extensive kerion forms.

while non-inflamed patches are present in others. Patients may be systemically ill with fever and regional lymphadenopathy.

It is thought that some patients have factors that predispose them to the development of a kerion, for example, whether or not the host is anergic to *Trichophyton*.

Carrier state. The 'carrier state' occurs primarily in adults exposed to infected children, but may also occur in children. The patient usually remains asymptomatic, but the dermatophyte can be cultured from the scalp. The infection can also present as a slight scale resembling dandruff or seborrhoeic dermatitis in adults and some children.

Diagnosis

Inflammatory changes in scalp infection are very variable. Apart from *T. tonsurans*, infections of anthropophilic origin cause significantly less inflammation than zoophilic or geophilic infections.

A kerion can be easily misdiagnosed as a bacterial abscess, and then inappropriately incised, drained and treated with antibiotics. Such treatment has no effect on the fungus and the infection will remain. The longer the infection remains, the greater the risk of scarring alopecia. It is important that any pustular eruption, particularly of the scalp, is recognized as a possible fungal infection and investigated accordingly. A number of infected hairs, ideally from non-inflammatory lesions, should be selected for examination as this increases the isolation rate. Hairs may be excised with a scalpel if they are subcutaneous. The choice of hairs may be assisted by examination with a Wood's lamp (see page 18). Early treatment with antifungal agents will hasten resolution of the infection, and consequently minimize residual scarring and alopecia. A history of direct or indirect animal contact is an important indicator of fungal infection in such cases.

Differential diagnosis. Although fungal infection is not the only cause of scaling patches of alopecia or scarring alopecia, it is always worth excluding because it is so easily treated. Other diseases that may cause a similar clinical picture include:
- alopecia areata
- trichotillomania (hair-pulling tics)
- seborrhoeic dermatitis
- psoriasis
- sebo-psoriasis and bacterial infection (e.g. impetigo, carbuncles, sycosis)
- folliculitis
- discoid lupus erythematosus
- lichen planus
- syphilis.

Favus

Favus is a specific form of tinea capitis caused only by *Trichophyton schoenleinii* (Figure 3.4). Favus is characterized by a significant degree of crusting and inflammation. The crust consists of a mixture of hyphae, neutrophils, epidermal cells and intertwined hair, which is known as a

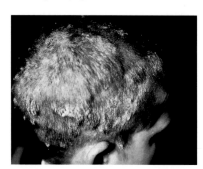

Figure 3.4 Favus caused by *Trichophyton schoenleinii*. This is a rare infection seen in restricted areas of the USA, north Africa and the Middle East.

scutulum, because of its characteristic cup shape. These crusts may cover the whole of the scalp, which consequently develops a yellowy-white appearance. Although the inflammatory response is significant, this is not a self-limiting infection, and follicular scarring and permanent alopecia are common sequelae. Favus is rare in the developed countries and tends to occur only in chronic care facilities, such as mental hospitals. In some parts of Africa, Asia and Latin America, however, the disease is still prevalent.

Treatment

Before the introduction of effective antifungal drugs, the only method of treatment was epilation, either by shaving or by X-ray therapy. The introduction of griseofulvin in the late 1950s proved, however, to be a watershed in the treatment of scalp infection. Although griseofulvin is only weakly fungistatic, it is highly effective in the treatment of most forms of tinea capitis and, as a result, such infection is now much less prevalent in the western world. In developing countries, a diagnosis is often unavailable or delayed and, even then, drug costs are often prohibitive.

New antifungal agents, notably the allylamines and triazoles, have the advantage that a shorter course of therapy is required than with griseofulvin, which increases compliance. However, these drugs cost significantly more than griseofulvin and, as a result, tinea capitis is likely to prove a continuing problem in the developing world for some time to come. Tinea capitis must be treated with an oral antimycotic (Table 3.1). Topical therapy is not effective.

Griseofulvin. All oral antifungal agents are effective in tinea capitis, but the gold standard is griseofulvin, 15 mg/kg/day of the ultramicrosize preparation or 20–25 mg/kg/day of the microsize suspension, continued for a minimum of 8 weeks. The ultramicronize particles are much smaller than the micronize ones, and allow for greater absorption. Doses may need to be adjusted to take this factor into account. For example, the current recommended dose for the liquid preparation, which is a microsize formulation, is 20–25 mg/kg/day, while that for the tablets, which contain the ultramicronize formulation, is 15 mg/kg/day. Many patients require therapy for more than 8 weeks and the general rule is to treat the patient until the hair starts regrowing and the fungal culture is negative.

TABLE 3.1

Antimycotic drugs used in the treatment of tinea capitis

	Dose	Treatment duration
Griseofulvin		
Microsize	20–25 mg/kg/day	8–12 weeks
Ultramicrosize	15 mg/kg/day	8–12 weeks
Terbinafine	10–20 kg body weight: 62.5 mg/day	1–4 weeks
	20–40 kg body weight: 125 mg/day	(> 6 weeks in
	> 40 kg body weight: 250 mg/day	*Microsporum canis* infections)
Itraconazole	Children: 5 mg/kg/day	4–6 weeks
	Adults: 200–400 mg/day	
Fluconazole	6 mg/kg/day	20 days
	5 mg/kg/day	4–6 weeks

Terbinafine is an excellent alternative to griseofulvin. The dose of terbinafine varies according to body weight (Table 3.1) and is usually given for 4 weeks, though some patients require treatment for only 1–2 weeks. *M. canis* infections acquired from cats or dogs, however, require treatment for 6 weeks or longer.

Itraconazole. A number of clinical trials have shown that itraconazole is very effective in the treatment of tinea capitis. In one study, involving 120 patients who had all been treated unsuccessfully with griseofulvin, in adults a switch to itraconazole 3–5 mg/kg/day for 4 weeks resulted in all patients being clinically and mycologically cured. Pulse-dosing with itraconazole is also effective. One hundred percent cure rates have been achieved in children with *Trichophyton tonsurans* infection when 1–3 weekly pulses were used, with 2–3 weeks off between pulses. Pulse-dosing is a reasonable option, considering the pharmacokinetic profile of itraconazole. In children, the capsule formulation of itraconazole precludes precise dosing, but a dose of as close to 5 mg/kg/day as possible should be taken with food or a cola beverage. The cyclodextrin solution formulation of itraconazole may prove beneficial in this situation.

Fluconazole is also effective in tinea capitis, though fewer data are available. One study has shown a dose of 6 mg/kg/day for 20 days to be effective. The availability of fluconazole in a pleasant-tasting liquid formulation that is already approved for use in children makes it an ideal substitute for griseofulvin in young children with tinea capitis who require a liquid formulation. In addition, fluconazole needs to be given for only 20 days, which further increases compliance.

Adjunctive therapy in tinea capitis includes the intermittent use of a 1–2% ketoconazole or selenium sulphide shampoo on a daily basis. All family members should receive treatment, because of the high transmission rate. Approximately 30% of adults exposed to a child with *T. tonsurans* tinea capitis acquire infection, albeit asymptomatically.

Because tinea capitis is highly contagious, a common dilemma is how to decide when the child can return to school. Oral antimycotic therapy and the use of an antifungal shampoo decrease the risk of transmission, and most authorities permit return to school after therapy has been initiated.

Prevention of tinea capitis

To prevent recurrent disease, it is important to check all family members for the possibility of tinea capitis. Many children develop a chronic infection due to re-exposure from a sibling, or even a parent. It is important to stress that **all** family members must use an antifungal shampoo, such as ketoconazole 2% or selenium sulphide, every day or every other day until the patient who is being treated is clinically and mycologically cured. A further month of treatment is recommended if the patient or family have been particularly recalcitrant. It is also important to emphasize that inanimate objects, such as combs, hairbrushes, barrettes and other hair accessories need to be discarded and/or disinfected. Boiling the comb or hair accessory in water for 5 minutes or more may be helpful, but it is preferable, in most instances, to discard such items, because fungal spores are so hard to destroy.

CHAPTER 4

Tinea corporis and cruris

Tinea corporis

Tinea corporis is dermatophytosis of the skin, excluding the hair and nails. All dermatophytes can cause tinea corporis and infection can occur anywhere on the body, though exposed skin is most commonly affected.

The clinical presentations of tinea corporis are diverse and may mimic many conditions. Skin changes may include the typical arcuate or annular pattern, circinate lesions, oval lesions, papulosquamous lesions, pustular and vesicular lesions, and occasionally granulomatous presentations (Figures 4.1–4.5). Not all rashes are generally annular, but most are generally scaly. The rash may not be scaly in a patient who has previously used a topical corticosteroid, but tinea corporis should always be considered when rashes fail to respond to such treatment. The extent of infection and inflammation may be affected by the particular pathogen, but is also mediated by the host immune response towards fungal antigens. Patients generally complain of itching, burning and/or pain.

The differential diagnoses include granuloma annulare, eczematous dermatoses, pityriasis rosea, psoriasis, parapsoriasis, discoid lupus and bacterial pyodermas.

Treatment. Topical therapy is generally effective in most patients with tinea corporis (Table 4.1). Patients should apply the topical agent to the affected skin and at least 2.5 cm around the advancing edge once or twice daily, or as recommended by the manufacturer. All the systemic antimycotics (Table 4.2) are effective in the treatment of tinea corporis and may be helpful as an adjunct to topical therapy. Systemic therapy is also indicated for extensive or widespread infection and chronic disease.

In general, it is important to avoid topical corticosteroids in the treatment of tinea corporis. Although their anti-inflammatory effect may reduce symptoms of itching, their use may potentially inhibit the cellular response to infection, promoting an exacerbation of inflammatory symptoms. Topical corticosteroids, including proprietary preparations containing a combination

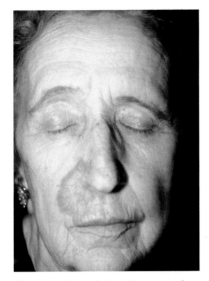

Figure 4.1 Tinea faciae. Ringworm of the face is uncommon, but may be difficult to recognize as it presents with erythema, scaling and sores.

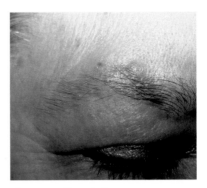

Figure 4.2 Tinea faciae.

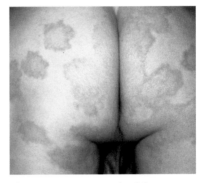

Figure 4.4 Tinea corporis of the buttocks.

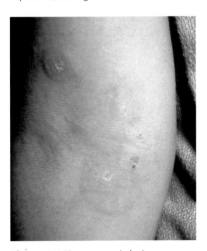

Figure 4.3 Tinea corporis lesions are annular, often irregular and may be multiple. It is often confused with other annular lesions such as eczema, annular erythemas or psoriasis.

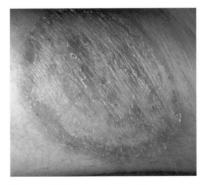

Figure 4.5 Tinea circinata of the arm. This is the classical ringworm lesion showing a round, inflamed rim with scaling in the centre.

31

TABLE 4.1

Topical antimycotic agents used in the treatment of cutaneous fungal infections

Azole family – imidazoles	Substituted pyridone derivative
• Clotrimazole	• Ciclopirox olamine
• Econazole	
• Ketoconazole	**Polyene drugs**
• Miconazole	• Nystatin
• Oxiconazole	• Amphotericin B
• Sulconazole	
	Miscellaneous
Allylamine family	• Tolnaftate
• Naftifine	• Selenium sulphide
• Terbinafine	• Whitfield's ointment
• Butinafine	• Zinc pyrithione

of a corticosteroid and an antimycotic agent, should particularly be avoided in the treatment of immunocompromised or diabetic patients.

Prevention. The treatment of tinea corporis is generally rewarding and effects a permanent cure. Identification of the causative pathogen may, however, provide useful information that may help to prevent re-exposure and reinfection. For example, patients who have been infected from an animal source, such as a kitten (*M. canis*), should have the animal treated appropriately by a veterinarian to prevent re-infection.

Whenever possible, contact with moist, damp environments, such as gymnasiums and locker rooms, should be avoided, as a high load of infective fungal elements from other people may be present.

Alternatively, the use of an antifungal shampoo (1% or 2% ketoconazole) and soap after exposure to these environments may help prevent infection. Tinea corporis also often results from close body contact with infected individuals, who should be identified and treated if possible. Patients should also be taught how to recognize and treat any sign of new or recurrent

infection promptly.

Tinea cruris

Tinea cruris is a common dermatophytic infection that occurs predominantly in men, but can occasionally develop in women. Infection occurs on the proximal thighs, crural folds and extends onto the buttocks (Figures 4.6 and 4.7).

A risk factor for tinea cruris is the presence of tinea pedis as inoculation of fungal elements from the foot onto clothing will spread the infection to a moist crural environment. As a result, men are more likely to develop tinea cruris than women, because the moist environment created by the scrotum increases the risk of infection. This area should be kept dry to reduce the likelihood of fungal infections. The intertriginous fold near the scrotum is usually the first site of involvement. The scrotal skin itself seems immune to infection and, if the scrotal skin is red or scaling, candidiasis, neurodermatitis, erythrasma, or another cutaneous disorder is more likely; this fact may be helpful in the differential diagnosis, particularly as erythrasma may mimic tinea cruris or occur concurrently with dermatophytic infection. Other risk factors for tinea cruris include obesity and diabetes mellitus.

It is also important to exclude *Candida* as a cause of a crural dermatosis. Women with a crural dermatosis are often infected with *Candida*, whereas men are significantly more likely to have a dermatophytic infection (see Table 8.1).

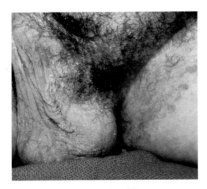

Figure 4.6 Tinea cruris. This presents with scaling in the groin extending onto the upper surface of the thigh and around the perineum.

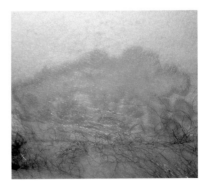

Figure 4.7 Tinea cruris.

TABLE 4.2

Systemic antimycotic agents for the treatment of cutaneous fungal infections

Drug	Dose and treatment duration	Indication
Griseofulvin	500–750 mg/day for 2–4 weeks	• Dermatophytes
Terbinafine	250 mg/day for 1 week	• Dermatophytes
Itraconazole	200 mg/day for 1 week	• Dermatophytes • *Candida* • *Pityrosporum* yeasts
Fluconazole	150 mg once a week for 2–4 weeks	• Dermatophytes • *Candida* • *Pityrosporum* yeasts
Ketoconazole	200 mg/day for 2–4 weeks	• Dermatophytes • *Candida* • *Pityrosporum* yeasts

Treatment. In most cases, treatment with topical antifungal agents is satisfactory, though patients with extensive disease may benefit from systemic therapy (Table 4.2). In addition, concomitant onychomycosis or tinea pedis should be treated (see pages 37 and 42).

When treating tinea cruris with an oral agent, it is important to bear in mind that only the azole family (ketoconazole, itraconazole and fluconazole) has activity against *Candida*; griseofulvin and terbinafine are unlikely to be of benefit in this situation.

Prevention. Recurrence of tinea cruris is common. One strategy to prevent recurrence is to instruct the patient to wear loose clothing and keep dry. The use of a topical powder that absorbs sweat may be helpful in many patients. In addition, the patient should be instructed to dry the crural area carefully after bathing and, if necessary, to use a hair dryer to thoroughly dry the genitalia and diminish any chance of moisture accumulation, which will predispose to fungal infection. A medicated absorbent powder should also be applied over the infected area. Reapplication of the powder during the day may help some patients. Obese patients may benefit from weight reduction.

CHAPTER 5
Tinea unguium (onychomycosis)

Onychomycosis is the most common cutaneous fungal infection in adults and probably occurs in about 10% of individuals. Infection is most common in the elderly. Most infected people are unaware of their infection and may believe that dystrophic nails are simply part of the ageing process. Patients should be made aware that the disease is contagious, and can be passed on to their friends and family members. Infection may be acquired from parents, schools, from gymnasium locker rooms or other public facilities. Those with untreated or partially treated plantar or interdigital fungal infection may eventually develop onychomycosis.

Epidemiology

Dermatophyte infection of nails affects the toenails in about 80% of cases and is likely to be one of the most common of dermatological diseases because of its chronicity. The disease has attracted much interest recently, largely because of the advent of more effective therapeutic agents. Various surveys have estimated the prevalence of onychomycosis at between 3 and 10% of the population depending upon the methodology of the survey. In any event, it is a very common condition and in all cases is preceded by relatively longstanding infection of the soles or toe clefts.

Presentation

There are four recognized clinical patterns of dermatophyte onychomycosis (Figures 5.1–5.4):

- distal and lateral subungual onychomycosis
- superficial white onychomycosis
- proximal subungual onychomycosis
- total dystrophic onychomycosis.

Distal and lateral subungual onychomycosis is the most common presentation and begins in the hyponichium of the distal and lateral edges of the nail. The disease initially affects only the nail bed and progresses proximally. Subungual hyperkeratosis develops leading to significant onycholysis, which eventually involves the whole of the nail bed. Secondary

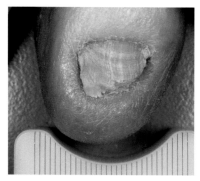

Figure 5.1 Tinea unguium. The entire nail plate has been infected and will crumble away.

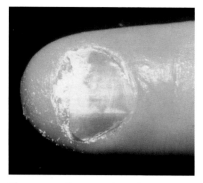

Figure 5.2 Tinea unguium showing fungal invasion of the distal and lateral portions of the nail plate.

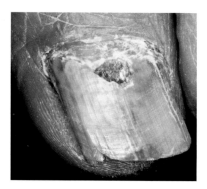

Figure 5.3 Tinea unguium. This is the proximal subungual form of the disease.

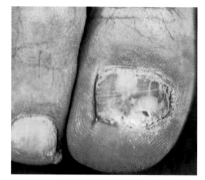

Figure 5.4 Tinea unguium, in which the whole nail plate is destroyed.

invasion of the nail plate is likely to occur, and the nail becomes friable and eventually breaks up, probably due to secondary trauma.

Superficial white onychomycosis is a disease of the surface of the nail plate and is much less common. It is mostly seen secondary to *T. mentagrophytes* infection.

Proximal subungual onychomycosis is rare. The disease begins at the proximal edge of the nail bed and is most often seen with concomitant disease, which may be systemic (e.g. AIDS) or local (e.g. peripheral vascular disease).

All three of these patterns of disease may eventually lead to total dystrophic onychomycosis, in which the whole of the nail bed and nail plate is involved. The pattern of infection is variable and occasionally pockets of tightly packed hyphae develop in the subungual space. The hyphae in such pockets are thick walled and somewhat abnormal, and constitute a dermatophytoma. In such cases, a dense creamy white area is seen beneath the nail, which is important because the infection may be relatively resistant to antifungal therapy without prior removal of the lesion. This appearance is most often seen in the great toenail.

The infected nail generally begins to lift up from the nail bed due to an accumulation of an excessive amount of debris (hyperkeratosis) under the nail. The nail will become yellow or brown and eventually quite thick, painful and difficult to cut. Infection can be confined to only one nail, but more commonly, several nails, on one or both feet are infected. Most patients have concurrent interdigital or moccasin tinea pedis, and some may also have tinea cruris. Most patients complain about nail discomfort, particularly when cutting, and many may experience pain during activities such as running, jogging, playing tennis and dancing.

Dermatophyte infection of the fingernails occurs in a similar pattern to the toenails, but it is much less common. It is very rare to see a patient with fingernail infection without toenail involvement.

Diagnosis of onychomycosis. Dermatophytes are responsible for onychomycosis in about 90% of all cases. Yeast infection occurs commonly in fingernails and non-dermatophyte moulds are nearly always secondary colonizers of previously damaged toenails. The primary cause of nail damage in such cases is most often a dermatophyte infection itself although other types of nail disease provide a convenient environment for saprophytic moulds. Non-dermatophyte moulds are most often 'diagnosed' by laboratories inexperienced in dealing with fungal specimens. The moulds grow faster than dermatophytes from a nail specimen and sometimes mask the dermatophyte altogether. A mistaken diagnosis of a non-dermatophyte mould infection is thus reported.

Treatment

Onychomycosis must be treated with an oral agent. Griseofulvin and ketoconazole are not generally used because of their low cure rates, high cost and risk of potential adverse events. The new antifungal agents, fluconazole, itraconazole and terbinafine, are all effective in onychomycosis, and are considered safe and well tolerated; ketoconazole is associated with hepatotoxicity. Cure rates with the newer antimycotics are also very acceptable and approach 80% in most patients. Higher cure rates can be obtained if the course of therapy is prolonged.

Itraconazole is generally given on a pulse or intermittent dosing schedule. A dose of 400 mg/day for 1 week/month for 3–4 consecutive months is the recommended regimen for patients with toenail infection. If only fingernail infection is present, a 2-month course or 1 week/month for 2 consecutive months is required. To avoid confusion, it is best to suggest that the patient takes the 1 week of therapy ('pulse') during the first week of each month; illustrating this regimen on a calendar may help to increase compliance. Note that itraconazole must be given with food to enhance absorption; a cola beverage and/or orange juice may also help absorption.

Fluconazole is generally administered at a dose of 150 mg once weekly for 6 months in toenail infection or 3 months in fingernail infection. Patients with very severe infection may require treatment for a longer period. Toenails grow very slowly (1 mm/month) and it therefore takes a year or more to grow out a healthy toenail.

Terbinafine. The allylamine, terbinafine, is also effective at a dose of 250 mg/day for 12 weeks continuously in toenail disease and 6 weeks continuously in fingernail disease.

Side-effects. Routine blood monitoring is not indicated with the new antifungal agents. Adverse events generally do not require discontinuation. Nausea and gastrointestinal disturbance are the most commonly experienced side-effects, but these can be allayed by taking the drug with food.

Rashes, such as a morbilliform eruption, may occasionally develop with any drug and generally require discontinuation and substitution of an unrelated drug. Fortunately, the patient may experience only minimal itching, which can be alleviated by topical steroids and anti-pruritic agents.

Prevention

Recurrence of onychomycosis may occur in some patients after discontinuation of therapy. *T. rubrum* is commonly found in hotel rooms, carpeting, gymnasiums, locker rooms and the floors of most public facilities. For this reason, it is essential that the importance of **always** wearing protective footwear to avoid re-exposure is emphasized to patients at risk. Other strategies (see Table 6.2, page 44) include application of an absorbent powder and antifungal powders containing miconazole, clotrimazole or tolnaftate in shoes and on feet, and wearing cotton, absorbent socks. It is also important to keep the nails as short as possible and to avoid sharing toenail clippers with friends and family members.

Shoes can contain a large number of infective fungal elements. In many instances, it is best to discard 'old and mouldy' footwear. If this is impossible, fungal elements can be eliminated by putting naphthalene mothballs in the shoes and leaving them in a tightly tied plastic bag for a minimum of 3 days. Afterwards, the patient can air the shoes to remove the odour of the naphthalene. The fungal spores should be dead. However, it is still helpful to continue to apply antifungal powders inside shoes to ensure that all infective fungal elements are eliminated.

An alternative is to spray a terbinafine solution into shoes on a periodic basis. Other infected family members should also be treated. Because both onychomycosis and tinea pedis are contagious, it does not make sense for only one member of a household to seek treatment because infection can be acquired from other infected members. It is also helpful to recommend comfortable shoes and to avoid trauma to the nail.

Candida **and onychomycosis.** It is important to discuss the role of nail salons to patients who develop nail infections. Frequent manicures and pedicures predispose many patients to the development of a variety of nail problems, including paronychial infections (infections around the nail fold), and primary onycholysis due to *Candida*, as well as dermatophytic nail infections. Patients who have developed these infections should be advised to frequent salons which employ a sterile technique.

It is important to avoid manipulation of the cuticle, which helps to prevent infection. Once the cuticle is damaged by dryness, manipulation, picking, or other activities, its ceases to function as a barrier and a variety of bacterial and fungal infections may ensue. Both the yeast, *Candida*, and bacteria (*Staphylococcus*, *Streptococcus* and *Pseudomonas*) are common nail pathogens. Paronychial infections present with swelling, tenderness and pus around the posterior or lateral nail fold, and may require oral antimycotic and/or antibiotic therapy. If *Candida* is implicated, ketoconazole, itraconazole or fluconazole are effective; fluconazole, 150 mg once weekly for approximately 3 months for fingernail and 6 months for toenail onychomycosis is effective in most patients. Other measures include soaking the affected nail in a disinfectant, application of topical antimycotic agents and the application of 4% thymol in chloroform or alcohol under or around the nailfold.

CHAPTER 6

Other tinea infections

Tinea imbricata

Tinea imbricata is caused by infection with *T. concentricum*. This organism produces a classic appearance of numerous concentric rings with pronounced peripheral scaling. Eventually, the entire trunk and extremities may be covered by this bizarre, but typical, eruption. It is a tropical disease that is seen only in Asia, the Pacific islands, and South and Central America. It generally runs a prolonged and chronic course, mainly because treatment is not readily available in endemic areas.

Treatment is essentially the same as for tinea corporis (see Chapter 4).

Tinea pedis

Tinea pedis refers to dermatophytosis of the foot, including the plantar surface and toe web space (Figures 6.1–6.4). There are four described presentations of tinea pedis: interdigital type, moccasin variety, inflammatory variety, and occasionally an ulcerative presentation of the

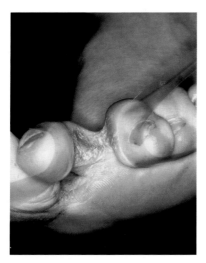

Figure 6.1 Tinea pedis, showing interdigital scaling.

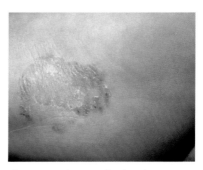

Figure 6.2 Tinea pedis, showing an inflammatory-type infection with blisters on the sole that is generally only seen with *Trichophyton interdigitale.*

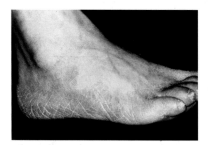 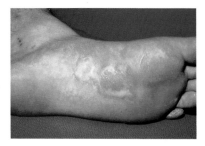

Figure 6.3 Moccasin tinea pedis, a chronic 'dry-type' of infection. The sole is covered with a dry, scaly rash, usually caused by *Trichophyton rubrum*.

Figure 6.4 Tinea pedis.

toe web. Interdigital tinea pedis is the most common and consists of dry, red, scaly toe webs. Moccasin tinea pedis is the most recalcitrant to therapy. The patients have chronic disease and nail infection is common adding to the recalcitrant nature. *T. rubrum* is the most common foot and nail pathogen. The entire plantar surface is dry and red. Inflammatory infections generally occur on medial foot, and vesicles or bullous lesions develop which are caused by one dermatophyte species – *T. mentagrophytes* – acquired from animal sources. Infections are generally self-limited. The ulcerative variety is quite rare and is generally a consequence of secondary bacterial infection in patients with interdigital tinea pedis who have other medical problems including peripheral vascular disease, diabetes mellitus, and/or immuno-deficiencies.

Treatment. Tinea pedis is treated with topical antifungal agents and oral antifungal agents may be given as adjunctive therapy. In patients who have extensive and hyperkeratotic moccasin tinea pedis, the addition of an exfoliant containing lactic acid or salicylic acid may help reduce scale and allow better penetration of the antifungal agent into the skin. Oral therapy (Table 6.1) is indicated in inflammatory or moccasin tinea pedis, and in the presence of onychomycosis. Both terbinafine and itraconazole are effective, as is fluconazole though fewer data to support its use in tinea pedis are available. Griseofulvin is of borderline effectiveness in most patients with tinea pedis, particularly in infection complicated by onychomycosis, and its use has been usurped by the newer agents.

TABLE 6.1

Oral treatment of tinea pedis

	Dose	Duration of treatment
Griseofulvin	500–1000 mg/day	1 month
Terbinafine	250 mg/day	1–2 weeks
Itraconazole	400 mg/day	1–2 weeks
Fluconazole	150 mg once a week	2–4 weeks
Ketoconazole	200 mg/day	2–4 weeks

Prevention. It is important to prevent re-exposure to the infective agent and to eliminate risk factors for recurrent disease. The simple strategies outlined in Table 6.2 can prevent the development of recurrent infection in most patients. However, some patients are inherently predisposed to infection and may require intermittent prophylactic therapy. Athletes participating in contact sports, military recruits and individuals who frequent health spas and gyms are especially at risk of recurrent infection. In these patients, the importance of proper foot hygiene must be emphasized.

Tinea manum

Hand infection is far less common than foot infection, but should always be suspected where a dry scaling eruption of one palm is seen (Figure 6.5). Scaling is particularly heavy in the skin creases. Fingernail involvement may also be present.

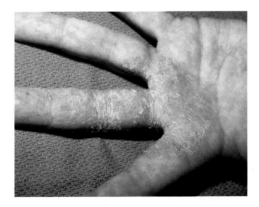

Figure 6.5 Tinea manum, a dry dermatophytosis, caused by *Trichophyton rubrum*, which affects the palms of the hands.

TABLE 6.2

Measures to prevent tinea pedis

- Use antibacterial soaps
- Dry feet thoroughly after bathing
- Liberally apply antifungal powders to feet after bathing
- Wear cotton socks to absorb sweat
- Change cotton socks frequently
- Wear protective footwear in hotels, locker rooms, gymnasiums and other public facilities
- Apply antifungal powders in shoes
- 'Rest' shoes periodically
- If recurrent disease appears, treat as quickly as possible

Treatment, again, is essentially the same as for tinea corporis (see Table 4.2). It often coexists with tinea pedis, and oral terbinafine and itraconazole are effective.

Prevention of tinea pedis is likely to prevent tinea manum.

CHAPTER 7
Pityriasis versicolor

Pityriasis (tinea) versicolor is caused by the yeast *M. furfur* (*P. orbiculare*). The adjective 'tinea' denotes infection with a dermatophyte and, therefore, is basically incorrect, but the name has been maintained because of tradition. A better name would be pityriasis versicolor, but this has not been uniformly accepted.

Epidemiology

Pityriasis versicolor is a common fungal infection that occurs predominantly in hot, humid climates. Infection is particularly common in the southern part of the USA and southern Europe, extending into the Mediterranean region, the Caribbean, Africa and South America. In some tropical regions, it is estimated that 50% of people are infected.

Presentation

Pityriasis versicolor is characterized by hypo- or hyperpigmented patches that tend to be fairly discrete, but can become confluent in widespread disease (Figures 7.1 and 7.2). In summer months, patients complain that their skin does not tan uniformly. In winter months, the skin may appear hyperpigmented, dryer and scalier. Pruritus is variable and occurs in some, but not all, patients. Generally, the rash is confined to the chest, back, and upper extremities, but occasionally, involvement of the lower extremities may be seen.

Figure 7.1 Pityriasis versicolor caused by the yeast *Malassezia furfur* (*Pityrosporum orbiculare*). The disease is characterized by multiple hypo- or hyperpigmented, ocasionally red, macules that are distributed across the upper trunk.

45

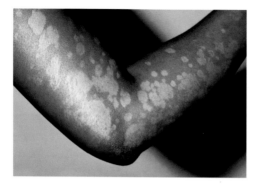

Figure 7.2 Pityriasis versicolor.

Pityrosporum folliculitis is characterized by itching follicular papules and pustules localized on the back, chest, upper arms, occasionally the neck and, more rarely, the face (Figure 7.3). It is associated with troublesome itching.

Treatment

Pityriasis versicolor is treated with topical (Table 7.1) or oral antimycotic agents.

Topical therapy. One of the more popular remedies for pityriasis versicolor is the use of 1–2% ketoconazole shampoo. The shampoo should be generously applied directly to the affected area and the patient instructed to leave the shampoo in contact with the skin for 10–15 minutes before washing it away. This should be repeated on a twice-weekly basis for 2–4 weeks to ensure complete eradication of the infection. Selenium sulphide shampoo can also be substituted, but the odour associated with this product may reduce compliance. All the topical azoles and allylamines

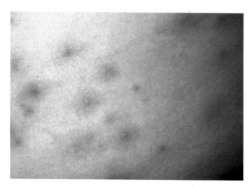

Figure 7.3 *Pityrosporum folliculitis* lesions, which appear on the back and upper trunk, occasionally on the neck and more rarely on the face.

TABLE 7.1

Topical antimycotic treatment effective in Pityriasis versicolor

- Selenium sulphide
- Ketoconazole shampoo
- Azole creams and lotions
- Allylamine creams and lotions
- Pyridone derivatives (ciclopirox olamine)
- Nystatin
- Topical amphotericin B
- 50% propylene glycol in water
- Zinc pyrithione (in dandruff shampoo)
- Salicylic acid preparations

applied once or twice daily to the affected area are also effective, though this may not be possible in patients with extensive infections. The development of terbinafine solution in a spray formulation is a convenient alternative to creams. Although effective, topical treatment may be associated with lower cure rates because of diminished compliance and, for this reason, an oral antimycotic is preferred by most patients.

After the infection has been appropriately treated, hyper- or hypopigmented patches may persist, representing postinflammatory hyper- or hypopigmentation. A mild topical corticosteroid may be used to help repigment the skin.

Oral therapy. Ketoconazole, 200 mg once daily for 5–7 days, is a simple, effective and satisfactory treatment for most patients. Alternatives include fluconazole, one dose of 400 mg continued once weekly for 2–3 weeks if necessary. Itraconazole, 200 mg/day for 3 consecutive days, may also be another excellent alternative. Oral griseofulvin and terbinafine are not effective in the treatment of pityriasis versicolor.

Prevention

Patients living in endemic regions are at high risk of recurrent disease. In these patients, using a ketoconazole shampoo as a 'soap' over the entire skin surface on a once-weekly basis may help to prevent infection. Patients at particularly high risk may require periodic administration of fluconazole or itraconazole, 200 mg once monthly, to prevent recurrent disease.

Pityriasis versicolor is not generally considered to be contagious. However, the application of oils to the skin, particularly those containing coconut oil, is a predisposing factor. It is, therefore, important to avoid the application of coconut-oil-based moisturizers, sunscreens and other products. Other natural oils, such as avocado and peanut oil, may also increase the risk of infection and should be avoided.

CHAPTER 8

Cutaneous *Candida* infections

Cutaneous candidiasis is caused predominantly by the yeast, *C. albicans*, though other species of *Candida* can occasionally cause infections. A number of risk factors predispose individuals to cutaneous *Candida* infections (Table 8.1).

Presentation

Cutaneous candidiasis occurs on the intertriginous regions of the axilla, under the breast, the panniculus and in the crural fold (Figures 8.1–8.3). The skin is typically bright red, moist and has satellite pustules.

Treatment

A variety of strategies are available for the treatment of cutaneous candidiasis. In the first instance, however, it is important to look for an underlying risk factor, such as exacerbation of diabetes, recent history of systemic antibiotic therapy or recent weight gain.

Topical antifungal agents are sufficient treatment in most patients with simple cutaneous candidiasis. The use of a drying agent, such as Burow's solution, may also be helpful in some situations.

TABLE 8.1

Risk factors for cutaneous candidiasis

- Diabetes mellitus
- Obesity
- Systemic antibiotic therapy
- History of vaginal candidiasis
- Use of oral contraceptives
- Use of spermicides (vaginal candidiasis)
- Residence in hot, humid climates
- Excessive sweating

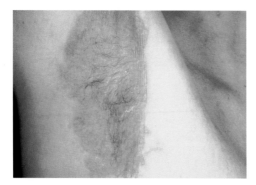

Figure 8.1 Cutaneous candidiasis of the axilla.

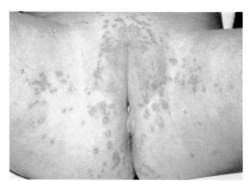

Figure 8.2 Cutaneous candidiasis of the thighs and groin. This irritant eczema is often secondarily infected with *Candida albicans*. The presence of yeasts may be suspected by the appearance of satellite pustules.

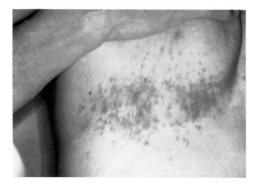

Figure 8.3 *Candida* intertrigo involving the skin under the breasts.

The addition of an antibacterial soap and the liberal application of drying powders or antifungal powders after bathing are helpful. It is also important to instruct the patient to keep the area as dry as possible and to use a hair dryer, if necessary, to dry the skin folds after bathing. This is especially helpful in obese patients with cutaneous candidiasis under a panniculus. Weight reduction would obviously also benefit these patients. One explanation for the development of infection at these sites is that the constant moist environment represents an optimum growth environment for *Candida*. In some patients, the skin is chronically damp from excess perspiration.

Oral antimycotic therapy includes fluconazole, 150 mg once weekly for 2 consecutive weeks, or itraconazole, 200 mg/day for up to 7 days. However, treatment should be continued until the infection has clinically resolved. Griseofulvin and terbinafine are not effective in patients with *Candida* infection.

Prevention

Cutaneous candidiasis can be prevented by keeping the skin as dry as possible, and by the liberal use of antifungal and absorbent powders. Patients with diabetes mellitus do best when blood sugars are maintained in an optimal range.

CHAPTER 9

Future trends

After decades of frustration and disappointment with the treatment and management of cutaneous fungal infections, physicians now have access to drugs with high cure rates and excellent safety profiles. Addition of the triazoles, itraconazole and fluconazole, and the allylamine, terbinafine, has been particularly beneficial, allowing reduced treatment durations and increased cure rates for most infections. Moreover, short treatment times improve patient compliance, reduce treatment costs and give patients hope that their often unsightly infections will be ended.

Accurate diagnosis

Perhaps the clinician's most important task is accurate diagnosis of the infection and determination of the fungal pathogen. To ensure this, both direct microscopy and fungal culture are necessary; direct microscopy will confirm the presence of a fungal pathogen immediately and culture will allow the organism to be identified. Because the newer antimycotics have different spectra of activity, different drugs may be required for different infections, making accurate determination of the pathogen more important than ever. Optimal antifungal treatment, which is effective against the infecting microorganism, is dependent on accurate diagnosis.

In the past decade, there have been significant advances in the development of effective and well-tolerated drugs for cutaneous mycotic disorders. What remains to be achieved? Unfortunately, many conditions, such as onychomycosis, tinea pedis and tinea capitis, are likely to remain diseases of modern civilization. Environmental factors that foster these fungal infections – longer life expectancies and increasing numbers of immunocompromised individuals – have combined to increase their prevalence. The recent availability of new antifungal agents with excellent safety profiles is battling against this trend.

In the near future, the area most deserving of our attention is improvement of diagnostic methods. Diagnostic methodology and fungal susceptibility testing lag behind therapeutic advances. We should turn our attention to these problems.

Key references

Aly R, Beutner KR, Maibach H, eds. *Cutaneous Infection and Therapy.* New York: Marcel Dekker, 1997.

Elewski BE, ed. *Cutaneous Fungal Infections.* 2nd edn. Oxford: Blackwell Science, 1998.

Evans EGV, Richardson MD, eds. *Medical Mycology: A Practical Approach.* Oxford: Oxford University Press, 1989.

Hay RJ. *Fungi and Skin Disease.* London: Gower Medical Publishing, 1993.

Jacobs PH, Nall L, eds. *Antifungal Drug Therapy: A Complete Guide for the Practitioner.* New York: Marcel Dekker, 1990.

Midgely G, Clayton YM, Hay RJ. *Diagnosis in Color: Medical Mycology.* Chicago: Mosby-Wolfe, 1997.

Richardson MD, Warnock DW. *Fungal Infection: Diagnosis and Management.* 2nd edn. Oxford: Blackwell Science, 1997.

Rippon JW, Fromtling RA, eds. *Cutaneous Antifungal Agents.* New York: Marcel Dekker, 1993.

Roberts DT, Evans EGV, Allen BR. *Fungal Infection of the Nail.* 2nd edn. London: Mosby-Wolfe Medical Communications, 1998.

Various authors. Terbinafine. *Rev Contemp Pharmacother* 1997;8:275–386.

Index

alopecia 24
arthrospore 7, 8, 9

'black-dot', in tinea capitis 24
Burow's solution 49

Candida albicans 7, 12
  in cutaneous candidiasis
  microscopical appearance 20
Candida intertrigo 49, 50
Candida paronychia 39
Candida species 7, 49
  in crural dermatosis 49
  culture 16
  in cutaneous candidiasis 49–51
  microscopical appearance 20
  in onychomycosis 39–40
  in paronychia 39
  response to antifungals 34
  see also Candida albicans
carrier state, tinea capitis 25
children, susceptibility 10
cutaneous candidiasis
  clinical presentation 49, 50
  prevention 51
  risk factors 49
  treatment 49–51

dermatophytes 7
  species 9
  transmission 9–10
diagnosis
  and clinical liaison 13–14
  culture 22
  microscopy 14, 17–21
  and patient information 17
  and specimen quality 15–16
  and specimen quantity 16–17

Epidermophyton floccosum 9

favus 26–7
fluconazole
  in cutaneous candidiasis 34, 51
  in pityriasis versicolor 47, 48
  in tinea capitis 28

in tinea corporis 34
in tinea cruris 34
in tinea pedis 43
in tinea unguium 38

griseofulvin
  in tinea capitis 27, 28
  in tinea corporis 34
  in tinea cruris 34
  in tinea pedis 42, 43

itraconazole
  in cutaneous candidiasis 34, 51
  in pityriasis versicolor 48
  in tinea capitis 28
  in tinea corporis 34
  in tinea cruris 34
  in tinea pedis 42, 43
  in tinea unguium 38

kerion 24–5
ketoconazole
  in cutaneous candidiasis 34
  shampoo
    in tinea capitis 28–9
    in pityriasis versicolor 46–7
  in tinea corporis 34
  in tinea cruris 34
  in tinea pedis 43

laboratory, role 13
lactic acid 42

Malassezia furfur 12
  microscopical appearance 20
  in pityriasis versicolor 45
Microsporum audouinii 9
  in tinea capitis 24
Microsporum canis 9, 10, 11
  microscopical appearance 21
  in tinea capitis 23, 24

onychomycosis
  Candida albicans in 39–40
  see also tinea unguium

paronychia 40
  clinical presentation 40
  treatment 40
*Pityrosporum orbiculare see
  Malassezia furfur*
pityriasis versicolor
  clinical presentation 45–6
  epidemiology 45
  prevention 47–8
  treatment 47–8
pityrosporum folliculitis 46

salicylic acid 42
Scytalidium dimidiatum 12
selenium sulphide, shampoo
  in tinea capitis 28–9
  in tinea corporis 32
shampoos
  in pityriasis versicolor 46, 47
  in tinea capitis 28–9
specimen
  collection 14–15, 16
  culture 22
  microscopical examination
    17–18, 20–1
  processing 18
  quality 15–16
  quantity 16–17

terbinafine
  in tinea capitis 27–8
  in tinea corporis 34
  in tinea pedis 43
  in tinea unguium 38
tinea capitis
  causal fungi 23
  clinical presentation 23–5
  diagnosis 25–6
  epidemiology 23
  prevention 29
  treatment 27–9
tinea corporis
  clinical presentation 30, 31
  prevention 32
  treatment 30–2

tinea cruris
  clinical presentation 33
  prevention 34
  treatment 34
tinea imbricata 41
tinea incognito 12
tinea manum
  clinical presentation 47
  prevention 44
  treatment 44
tinea pedis
  clinical presentation 41–2
  prevention 43, 44
  treatment 42–3
tinea unguium
  diagnosis 37
  epidemiology 35
  prevention 39–40
  treatment 37–8
Trichophyton species 9
Trichophyton concentricum 41
Trichophyton equinum 10, 11
Trichophyton erinacea 10, 11
Trichophyton gourvilli 23
Trichophyton interdigitale 9, 41
Trichophyton mentagrophytes
  42
  arthrospores of 8
  growth on hair 9
  growth on nail 7–9
  growth on skin 7–9
  in tinea capitis 23
Trichophyton mentagrophytes
  var. *interdigitale* 9
Trichophyton mentagrophytes
  var. *mentagrophytes* 9
Trichophyton rubrum 9
  culture 22
  in tinea capitis 23
  in tinea pedis 42
Trichophyton schoenleinii 26–7
Trichophyton soudense 23
Trichophyton verrucosum 9, 10,
  11, 24
Trichophyton violaceum 23
Trichophyton tonsurans 23, 24,
  25
  microscopical appearance 21

Other titles available in the *Fast Facts* series

Anxiety, Panic and Phobias
by Malcolm H Lader and Thomas W Uhde

Allergic Rhinitis
by Niels Mygind and Glenis K Scadding

Benign Prostatic Hyperplasia (third edition)
by Roger S Kirby and John D McConnell

Coeliac Disease
by Geoffrey Holmes and Carlo Catassi

Contraception
by Anna Glasier and Beverly Winikoff

Diseases of the Testis
by Timothy J Christmas, Michael D Dinneen and Larry Lipshultz

Dyspepsia
by Michael J Lancaster Smith and Kenneth L Koch

Endometriosis
by Hossam Abdalla and Botros Rizk

Epilepsy
by Martin J Brodie and Steven C Schachter

Headaches
by Richard Peatfield and J Keith Campbell

Hyperlipidaemia
by Paul Durrington and Allan Sniderman

Irritable Bowel Syndrome
by Kenneth W Heaton and W Grant Thompson

Menopause
by David H Barlow and Barry G Wren

Stress and Strain
by Cary L Cooper and James Campbell Quick

Urinary Continence
by Julian Shah and Gary Leach

To order, please contact:

Health Press Limited
Elizabeth House, Queen Street,
Abingdon, Oxford OX14 3JR, UK
Tel: +44 (0)1235 523233
Fax: +44 (0)1235 523238
Email: post@healthpress.co.uk

Or visit our website:
www.healthpress.co.uk

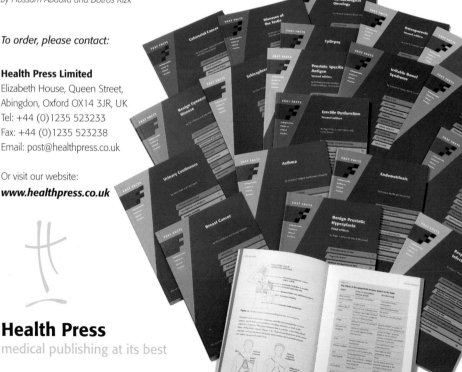

Health Press
medical publishing at its best